NOTES TO ASK THE DR:

_____

_____

_____

_____

_____

_____

_____

_____

_____

www.FamilyChiropractor.com

TABLE OF CONTENTS

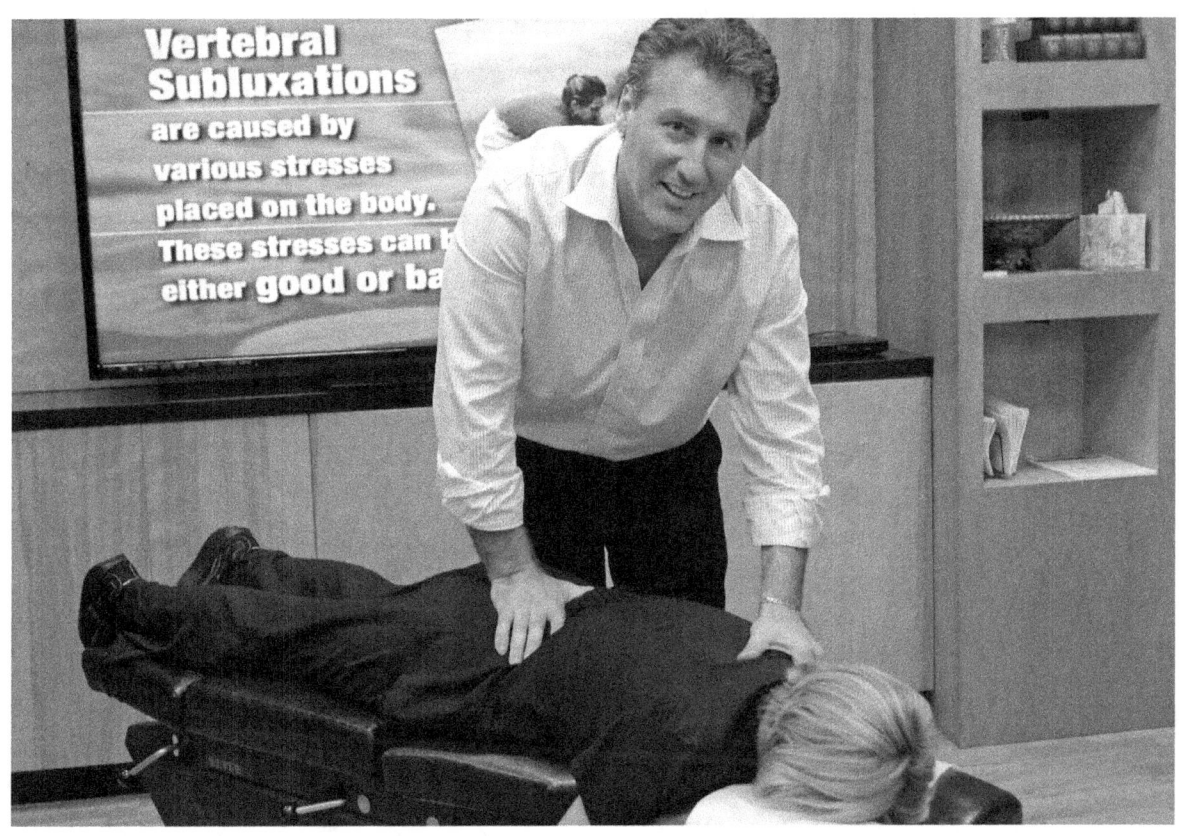

Chiropractic is the second largest of the three primary health care provider segments in the United States. Dr. Brent Baldasare and his wife Angela founded Affinity Health & Wellness Center in 2000.

INTRODUCTION

"My office was born out of a life-long passion to help people. As a victim of a paralyzing injury I know the importance of having a compassionate doctor and team to assist in getting back to top physical, chemical and emotional health. I am here to serve. If we can't help you we'll find someone that can." - Dr. Brent Baldasare

We are so happy that your journey to wellness has led you to try chiropractic care. As chiropractors our philosophy is simple, yet profound. As a profession, the primary belief is in natural and conservative methods of health care. Doctors of chiropractic have a deep respect for the human body's ability to heal itself without the use of surgery or medication.

We devote careful attention to the biomechanics, structure and function of the spine, its effects on the musculoskeletal and neurological systems, and the role played by the proper function of these systems in the preservation and restoration of health. A Doctor of chiropractic is one who is involved in the treatment and prevention of disease, as well as the promotion of public health, and a wellness approach to patient healthcare.

My personal journey began as a result of a paralyzing football injury that left me with two choices. The first choice was to have spinal surgery and the second was to find an alternative that would relieve the pressure to the nerves that supplied function to my legs.

On the recommendation of my trainer I tried chiropractic and twenty years to this day I've never had surgery and regained full use of my legs. I know I'm truly blessed and I'm not suggesting chiropractic is a cure all for paralysis but I am a walking testament that there is a powerful healing force in the body that if given the proper neurological, emotional and nutritional channels can perform miraculous healing.

Let us share with you a brief introduction to the profession that chose me.

1

A BACKGROUND OF CHIROPRACTIC CARE

The world's understanding of the efficacy of chiropractic care is still in its early stages even though knowledge of chiropractic science has been around to some degree as long as recorded time. Early chiropractors were jailed and they were publicly mocked by the medical community as charlatans and quacks. Until a brave group of doctors took on the powerful AMA and exposed an illegal conspiracy to destroy chiropractic. Here is a brief summary of the result.

Summary of Judge's Opinion and Order

On August 27, 1987, Judge Susan Getzendanner, United States District Judge for the Northern District of Illinois Eastern Division, found the American Medical Association, The American College of Surgeons, and The American College of Radiology, guilty of having conspired to destroy the profession of chiropractic in the United States. In a 101-page opinion, Judge Getzendanner ruled that the American Medical Association and its co-conspirators had violated the Sherman Antitrust Laws of the United States. Judge Getzendanner ruled that they had done this by organizing a national boycott of doctors of chiropractic by medical physicians and hospitals using an ethics ban on interprofessional cooperation.

Evidence at the trial showed that the defendants took active steps, often covert, to undermine chiropractic educational institutions, conceal evidence of the usefulness of chiropractic care, undercut insurance programs for patients of chiropractors, subvert government inquiries into the efficacy of chiropractic, engage in a massive misinformation campaign to discredit and destabilize the chiropractic profession and engage in numerous other activities to maintain a medical physician monopoly over health care in this country.

A HISTORY OF CHIROPRACTIC CARE

Its history begins at least as far back as recorded history with the healers of those times aware of a connection between the health of the spine and the health of the individual. It continues into the modern world where chiropractors are put through extensive training to be licensed to diagnose and treat problems within the body.

"The roots of chiropractic care can be traced all the way back to the beginning of recorded time. Writings from China and Greece written in 2700 B.C. and 1500 B.C. mention spinal manipulation and the manoeuvring of the lower extremities to ease low back pain. Hippocrates, the Greek physician, who lived from 460 to 357 B.C., also published texts detailing the importance of chiropractic care." In one of his writings he declares, "Get knowledge of the spine, for this is the requisite for many diseases".

In 1895, Daniel David Palmer delivered the first chiropractic adjustment to Harvey Lillard, a janitor in his office. Harvey had been deaf since injuring his back in a childhood accident. Harvey had a full recovery, including the restoration of his hearing, after that one adjustment.

Chiropractic is hands on healing. The healing process is started through manipulation of the spine or extremity that has lost its ability to function correctly. The natural alignment of the bones allows for optimal blood flow and nerve conduction and increases the ability of the immune system to ward off illness.

Chiropractors are the only doctors that are specifically trained to restore spinal balance. No other doctor or profession makes this claim. The emphasis of chiropractic is that the body heals itself, it's never the Band-Aid® that heals the cut, and it's never the pill that cures the cold.

The body, when functioning properly, heals and maintains itself. It's our job as chiropractors to remove any nerve interference that the body is experiencing so that the body can do its job: maintain your health!

*The word Chiropractic is a combination of two Greek words: **cheiros** means hand, and **prakikos** means practice. This combination is frequently interpreted to mean "**done by hand**."*

Throughout the twentieth century, doctors of chiropractic gained legal recognition in all fifty states. A continuing recognition and respect for the chiropractic profession in the United States has led to growing support for chiropractic care all over the world.

The research that has emerged from "around the world" has yielded incredibly influential results, which have changed, shaped and molded perceptions of chiropractic care. The report, *Chiropractic in New Zealand* published in 1979 strongly supported the efficacy of chiropractic care and elicited medical cooperation in conjunction with chiropractic care.

The 1993 *Manga* study published in Canada investigated the cost effectiveness of chiropractic care. The results of this study concluded that chiropractic care would save hundreds of millions of dollars annually with regard to work disability payments and direct health care costs.

Even more recent research from Dr. Haaviks new book called The Reality Check reveals how receiving chiropractic adjustments on a regular basis for as little as a few months can actually change the way our brain functions. By adjusting into the small joints and muscles of the spine it can actually help reboot how the data is processes to the brain.

She uses the metaphor of a computer that runs slow because it has to many programs open that are continuously draining the resources of the computer. By restarting the computer it clears out unnecessary data and it runs better. The same holds true for how these small muscle spindles near the spine continuously tell our brain where and what position the body is in. If they are over or under stimulated the brain receives inaccurate information that can lead to a whole host of functional problems such as headaches, pain and poor mobility.

EDUCATIONAL REQUIREMENTS FOR CHIROPRACTORS

According to the American Chiropractic Association the educational requirements for doctors of chiropractic are among the most stringent of any of the health care professions.

The typical applicant at a chiropractic college has already acquired nearly four years of pre-medical undergraduate college education, including courses in biology, inorganic and organic chemistry, physics, psychology and related lab work. Once accepted into an accredited chiropractic college, the requirements become even more demanding — four to five academic years of professional study are the standard. Because of the hands-on nature of chiropractic, and the intricate adjusting techniques, a significant portion of time is spent in clinical training.

Doctors of chiropractic — who are licensed to practice in all 50 states, the District of Columbia, and in many nations around the world — undergo a rigorous education in the healing sciences, similar to that of medical doctors. In some areas, such as anatomy, physiology, and rehabilitation, they receive more intensive education than most medical doctors or physical therapists.

Curriculum Requirements For the Doctor of Chiropractic Degree (DC) in comparison to the Doctor of Medicine Degree (MD) and the Doctor of Physical Therapy Degree (DPT) [1,2]

	Average Program Length	Average Classroom and Clinical Study Hours Prior to Graduation*	Advanced Certification Available
Chiropractic Curriculum	4 years	4,820	Yes
Medical Curriculum	4 years	4,670	Yes
Physical Therapy Curriculum	3 years	3,398	Yes

* Does not include hours attributed to post-graduation residency programs.

Like other primary health care doctors, chiropractic students spend a significant portion of their curriculum studying clinical subjects related to evaluating and caring for patients.

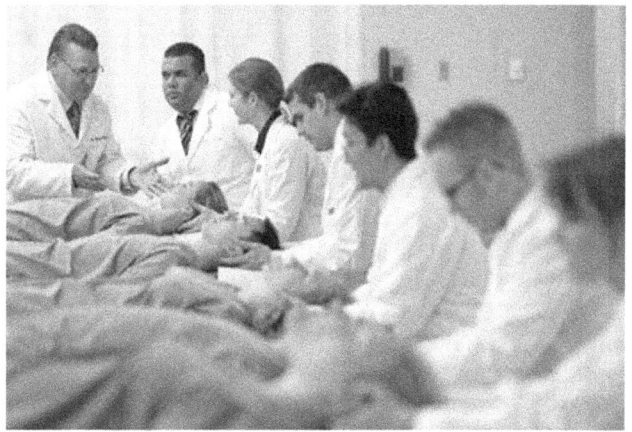

Typically, as part of their professional training, they must complete a minimum of a one-year clinical-based program dealing with actual patient care. In total, the curriculum includes a minimum of 4,200 hours of classroom, laboratory and clinical experience. The course of study is approved by an accrediting agency which is fully recognized by the U.S. Department of Education. This has been the case for more than 25 years.

Before they are allowed to practice, doctors of chiropractic must pass national board examinations and become state-licensed. Chiropractic colleges also offer post-graduate continuing education programs in specialty fields ranging from sports injuries and occupational health to orthopedics and neurology. These programs allow chiropractors to specialize in a healthcare discipline or meet state re-licensure requirements.

This extensive education prepares doctors of chiropractic to diagnose health care problems, treat the problems when they are within their scope of practice and refer patients to other health care practitioners when appropriate.

References
1- Meeker W, Haldeman H. Chiropractic: A Profession at the Crossroads of Mainstream and Alternative Medicine. Annals of Internal Medicine 2002, Vol 136, No 3.
2- American Physical Therapy Association. 2005-2006 Fact Sheet, Physical Therapist Education Programs. January 2007.

2

WHAT IS

CHIROPRACTIC CARE?

What is chiropractic care? Is it effective? Who can benefit from chiropractic care? All these questions are at the forefront of a patient's mind when he or she considers chiropractic treatment as an option.

Chiropractic is a health care profession that focuses on disorders of the musculoskeletal system and the nervous system, and the effects of these disorders on general health. Chiropractic care is used most often to treat neuro-musculoskeletal complaints, including but not limited to back pain, neck pain, pain in the joints of the arms or legs, and headaches.

Doctors of Chiropractic – often referred to as chiropractors or chiropractic physicians – practice a drug-free, hands-on approach to health care that includes patient examination, diagnosis and treatment. Chiropractors have broad diagnostic skills and are also trained to recommend therapeutic and rehabilitative exercises, as well as to provide nutritional, dietary and lifestyle counseling.

The most common therapeutic procedure performed by doctors of chiropractic is known as "spinal manipulation," also called "chiropractic adjustment."   The purpose of manipulation is to restore joint mobility by manually applying a controlled force into joints that have become hypomobile – or restricted in their movement – as a result of a tissue injury. Tissue injury can be caused by a single traumatic event, such as improper lifting of a heavy object, or through repetitive stresses, such as sitting in an awkward position with poor spinal posture for an extended period of time. In either case, injured tissues undergo physical and chemical changes that can cause inflammation, pain, and diminished function for the sufferer. Manipulation, or adjustment of the affected joint and tissues, restores mobility, thereby alleviating pain and muscle tightness, and allowing tissues to heal.

Chiropractic adjustment rarely causes discomfort. However, patients may sometimes experience mild soreness or aching following treatment (as with some forms of exercise) that usually resolves within 12 to 48 hours.

In many cases, such as lower back pain, chiropractic care may be the primary method of treatment. When other medical conditions exist, chiropractic care may complement or support medical treatment by relieving the musculoskeletal aspects associated with the condition.

Doctors of chiropractic may assess patients through clinical examination, laboratory testing, diagnostic imaging and other diagnostic interventions to determine when chiropractic treatment is appropriate or when it is not appropriate. Chiropractors will readily refer patients to the appropriate health care provider when chiropractic care is not suitable for the patient's condition, or the condition warrants co-management in conjunction with other members of the health care team.

A few interesting facts about back pain:
- Low back pain is the single leading cause of disability worldwide, according to the Global Burden of Disease 2010.
- One-half of all working Americans admit to having back pain symptoms each year.[2]
- Back pain is one of the most common reasons for missed work. In fact, back pain is the second most common reason for visits to the doctor's office, outnumbered only by upper-respiratory infections.
- Most cases of back pain are mechanical or non-organic—meaning they are not caused by serious conditions, such as inflammatory arthritis, infection, fracture or cancer.
- Americans spend at least $50 billion each year on back pain—and that's just for the more easily identified costs.[3]
- Experts estimate that as many as 80% of the population will experience a back problem at some time in our lives.[4]

1. Jensen M, Brant-Zawadzki M, Obuchowski N, et al. Magnetic Resonance Imaging of the Lumbar Spine in People Without Back Pain. N Engl J Med 1994; 331: 69-116.

2. Vallfors B. Acute, Subacute and Chronic Low Back Pain: Clinical Symptoms, Absenteeism and Working Environment. Scan J Rehab Med Suppl 1985; 11: 1-98.

3. This total represents only the more readily identifiable costs for medical care, workers compensation payments and time lost from work. It does not include costs associated with lost personal income due to acquired physical limitation resulting from a back problem and lost employer productivity due to employee medical absence. In Project Briefs: Back Pain Patient Outcomes Assessment Team (BOAT). In MEDTEP Update, Vol. 1 Issue 1, Agency for Health Care Policy and Research, Rockville,

4. In Vallfors B, previously cited.

THE SCIENCE BEHIND CHIROPRACTIC CARE

Everyone has that image from television, movies, and possibly real chiropractic experiences of a chiropractor cracking a patient's back, but what does this really do? How does correcting the positioning of the spine affect the body in any appreciable way? To grasp the purpose of spinal realignment, you must first understand the basic way in which the body works and how the brain and the rest of the body are connected.

Think of the basic science of the body. The brain is the start of it all. The brain sends out a signal every time a part of the body needs to do anything. If you want to lift your arm then the brain sends a signal down to your arm to tell it to move. If there is food in your stomach then the brain sends a signal to tell your stomach to produce digestive juices. If your brain is going to know what is going on in the body so that it can send out the appropriate signals then it has to be able to receive signals back from the body as well.

This is clearly an oversimplified explanation but more than adequate to illustrate the following point. The brain sends signals for the production of neurotransmitters, the operation of various organs, the secretion of digestive juices, and everything else that goes on in the body basically, but how do these messages get where they are going?

They are sent through the spinal cord and then down the spinal nerves. The nerves are the route that these messages take to make their way to various parts of the body so that they can be received and carried out. A spine that is in perfect health and that is perfectly aligned allows for an unobstructed pathway through which these signals from the brain can be transmitted.

If, however, the spine is not in proper alignment then these signals cannot travel as efficiently or even as effectively to their chosen destinations. Orders sent from the brain may not be carried out as quickly or as effectively. In severe cases, they may not be carried out at all.

Since chiropractic's inception in 1895 there has been an understanding of the crucial relationship between the integrity of the spinal column and the function of the nerve system as a whole and specifically the tissues and organs that they supply. The interrelatedness of the spine and nervous system, even way back then, was evident in its simplest of understandings.

It was this basic observation that led to the profession of chiropractic focusing on the function of the nervous system and how it is the main source for transmitting the inborn intelligence and information one requires to express their fullest health potential. In essence, to the degree one maintained a healthy nervous system, one free of interference and aberrant communication in relation to the spine, is to the degree one was able to express the fullest potential for life and health.

Chiropractors influence the function of the nerve system through the spine and spinal subsystems thereby allowing the body to increase its own inborn ability to sef-regulate and self-heal.

Why Don't Some M.D.s Recognize the Importance of Nerve Function?

Fast forward 110 years later. I can't tell you how many times I have a person in front of me to whom I explain these simple workings of the importance of nerve function in the role of their health. I know I am not the only chiropractor who hears this next line all too frequently, *"Why didn't my M.D. tell me that?"*

Vitalism is the doctrine that "living organisms are fundamentally different from non-living entities because they contain some non-physical element or are governed by different principles than are inanimate things".

My answer is usually something along the lines of, "Maybe they just simply don't know and you should explain it to them." In truth I do not know the answer, but my best guess would be that their understandings are based on a medical, mechanistic view – instead of a holistic or vitalistic philosophy.

There is sometimes a professional biasness that chiropractic ideas have not come from any medical research or any allopathic physician and therefore are not valid.

Well thanks to an early pioneering Medical Doctor who spent many long hours in the lab we have results that support the basics of the chiropractic view of a life and death relationship between the nerves and the function of the organs as they relate to the spine.

They are called: **The Winsor Autopsies**

Henry Winsor, a medical doctor in Haverford, Pennsylvania, asked the question: "Chiropractors claim that by adjusting one vertebra, they can relieve stomach troubles and ulcers; by adjusting another, menstrual cramps; and by adjusting others conditions such as kidney diseases, constipation, heart disease, thyroid conditions, and lung disease may resolve–but how?"

Dr. Winsor decided to investigate this new science and art of healing, called chiropractic. After graduating from medical school, Dr. Winsor was inspired by chiropractic and osteopathic literature to experiment. He planned to dissect human and animal cadavers to see if there was indeed a relationship between any diseased internal organ discovered on autopsy and the vertebrae associated with the nerves that went to the organ. As he wrote:

"The object of these necropsies (dissections) was to determine whether any connection existed between minor curvatures of the spine, on the one hand, and diseased organs on the other; or whether the two were entirely independent of each other."

The University of Pennsylvania gave Dr. Winsor permission to carry out his experiments. In a series of three studies he dissected a total of 75 human and 22 cat cadavers. The following are Dr. Winsor's results:

"Two hundred twenty-one structures other than the spine were found diseased. Of these, 212 were observed to belong to the same sympathetic (nerve) segments as the vertebrae in curvature. Nine diseased organs belonged to different sympathetic segments from the vertebrae out of line.

These figures cannot be expected to exactly coincide ... for an organ may receive sympathetic filaments from several spinal segments and several organs may be supplied with sympathetic (nerve) filaments from the same spinal segments. In other words, there was nearly a 100% correlation between minor curvatures of the spine and diseases of the internal organs.

The Diseases examined:

Stomach Diseases: All nine cases of spinal misalignment in the mid-thoracic area (T5-T9) had stomach disease.

Lung Disease: All 26 cases of lung disease had spinal misalignments in the upper thoracic spine.

Liver Disease: All 13 cases of liver disease had misalignments in the mid thoracic (T5-T9)

Gallstones: All five cases with gallstone disease had spinal misalignments in the mid thoracic.

Pancreas: All three cases with pancreas disease had spinal misalignments in the mid thoracics.

Spleen: All 11 cases with spleen diseases had spinal misalignments in the mid thoracics.

Kidney: All 17 cases with kidney disease were out of alignment in the lower thoracics.

Prostate and Bladder Disease: All eight cases with kidney, prostate and bladder disease had the lumbar (L2-L3) vertebrae misaligned

Uterus: The two cases with the uterine conditions had the second lumbar misaligned.

Heart Disease: All 20 cases with heart and pericardium conditions had the upper five thoracic vertebrae (T1-T5) misaligned.

Dr. Winsor's results are published in The Medical Times, November 1921, and are found in any medical library. That's right this has been known since 1921!

3

WHAT DO CHIROPRACTORS DO EXACTLY?

While visiting a chiropractor is similar to visiting other healthcare providers, it does have some unique elements. You will likely find the office setting and intake procedures quite familiar, but many notice the distinctive appearance of the chiropractic treatment table. These tables are often quite elaborate to allow specific positioning and movement during spinal adjustments and thus assist the chiropractic treatment.

What happens during the physical exam?

We usually start with a routine physical exam, then follow it with an exam that focuses on the spine, with particular attention given to the areas of complaint. We will most likely examine your whole spine. For example, if you had a low back complaint, we would also likely perform a neck exam because the adaptations resulting from injury or misalignments in one area can result in secondary irritations somewhere else in the spine.

Most often, we will take X-rays of your spine prior to treatment. The purpose of the X-rays is to study the condition of the bony anatomy and soft tissues. It also helps us understand the extent of wear, any anomalies in your spine, and other factors that will guide us in the development of a corrective treatment plan.

The physical exam typically includes a variety of assessments, such as range of motion tests, palpation, reflex testing, muscle strength comparisons, and neurological and orthopedic tests focused on the main complaint.

What goes into a treatment plan?

Following the assessments, we will develop a treatment plan that takes into account:

- The extent of your injury or irritation
- Your general health
- The condition of your spine as affected by age and previous injury
- What your goals are - this is most important item

Your goals of treatment should result from the discussion you have with your chiropractor. Many people seek simple relief of pain or discomfort, while others want to begin a regimen of ongoing care meant to improve their general health. In initial consultations, your chiropractor will tell you the status of your condition and recommend an approach to care. Ask questions. As in any professional-patient relationship, trust and mutual understanding are vitally important.

What is a typical treatment?

"Adjustments" are the central part of chiropractic treatment. The chiropractic adjustment is a specific therapeutic manipulation that uses controlled force, leverage, direction, amplitude, and velocity directed at specific joints. In other words, an adjustment involves a lot more than just "cracking your back".

Your chiropractor will most often make these adjustments to the spine, but he or she might adjust other joints, such as the ankle, knee, wrist, elbow, or shoulder in order to restore structural alignment or to improve joint function. Again, proper structure is necessary for proper function, and proper extremity function is an important part of healthy daily living.

THE TRUTH ABOUT ADJUSTMENTS

You might wonder if a patient will feel pain while these adjustments are being performed. The majority of patients will not. There may be some slight discomfort initially as they adjust to the treatment process, but this is minor and will pass. Actually, many patients report a rapid sensation of relief following adjustments for the conditions that they seek treatment for.

As stated earlier, the chiropractor does not merely seek to treat the condition that a patient came in for but checks for any misalignments that may be present. This way any possible problems or positioning that could lead to future problems are all treated. The treatment is not limited to attempts at treating the problem at hand.

In fact, it is not uncommon for patients to experience an improvement in symptoms that they thought were unrelated to their original complaint or just in their overall feeling of well being. The integrated nature of the body and the way that the spine influences the body as a whole makes this a very real occurrence.

Adjustments may be used to deal with acute conditions, chronic conditions, or they may be used as more of a preventative measure. A patient does not necessarily need to wait until a problem is fully developed before seeking out treatment for spinal misalignment. Developing or potential conditions may be caught early and rectified before they can come to fruition. Also, the general health and feeling of well being may be improved through chiropractic intervention even if there is not one discernable problem to treat. Because of the all inclusive nature of spinal health, preventative chiropractic adjustments are quite beneficial for many patients.

During the course of a session, your chiropractor introduces the appropriate amount of pressure using their hands to the patient's body to complete each adjustment. This is where the extensive curriculum that a chiropractor undergoes when training pays off. These somewhat simple movements require a comprehensive background in physiology and related subjects to be performed correctly and safely.

A patient may find it disconcerting to hear a loud cracking or popping noise coming from joints as adjustments are made. This sound is created by small amounts of gas (Nitrogen) being moved about the joints during the adjustments. The movement of the gas creates the sound. This sound may not always be present when an adjustment is made and is not an indication of the efficacy of the treatment.

It is similar to a person cracking their knuckles. The release of the gas creates the cracking sound and does not necessarily indicate anything more that the movement of the gas.

The amount of force required to complete an adjustment is not the same from one patient to the next. The amount of pressure necessary to perform the appropriate spinal adjustment depends largely on the person and the adjustment to be made.

If the problems are concentrated in the neck then a chiropractor may focus efforts in that area. Cervical adjustments are utilized to free up the neck joints, relieving the tension that may be present and aiding the mobility of the muscles.

Clearly, neck adjustments are not likely to require as much force as adjustments performed on the lower parts of the spine. It is the chiropractor's training that allows for the assessment of the situation and the application of the correct amount of force.

Although the popularized image of chiropractic care may be one that includes a loud cracking or popping sound, the force applied varies and is highly controlled. The amount of force necessary to create changes in one person may be too much for another and what is the right amount of force for another person may not be sufficient for yet another. The treatment, while consistent, is individualized.

Chiropractors require the physical strength to make the necessary adjustments. The amount of strength needed may vary depending on the individual patient and the adjustments that are necessary. The physicality of this profession is another prerequisite for chiropractors. We have to not only know how to perform the adjustments but be physically able to complete them as well.

The treatments are not intended to cause the patient any pain although they may result in a feeling of soreness for a patient. This soreness is often likened to the feeling a person has after an exercise session.

Some patients may wonder if they are able to perform adjustments on themselves. Often individuals can create a similar popping sound with their joints if they try. This is not advisable. Chiropractic adjustments are precise and require years of study to perform correctly. The creation of this popping or cracking sound is not an indication that anything is being accomplished and is certainly not an indication that anything is being done correctly. Such movements may not be doing anything or may be creating adverse effects. Adjustments should always be performed by trained professionals.

The question of safety will likely arise when discussing adjustments. Knowing that the spine is a sensitive and essential part of the body, one would rightly wonder if manipulating it in this manner is safe. Clearly, the nature of chiropractic adjustments does introduce an element of risks just as any treatment protocol would.

Chiropractic care is recognized for being safe, medication free, and a non-invasive way of correcting problems caused by improper spinal alignment. Chiropractic care has a track record for being one of the safest methods of treatment in healthcare. This is evident by the extremely low malpractice insurance rates chiropractors incur verses medical doctors.

PREGNANT WOMEN

A special case is that of pregnant women. Patients may wonder if chiropractic care can be administered when a woman is pregnant. The improved functioning of the body is advantageous for anyone. Because chiropractic care is individualized, the proper adjustments and amount of pressure are evaluated on a patient to patient basis and are therefore adjusted to any special needs of a patient, including pregnancy.

Pregnant women who receive chiropractic treatments often report that the delivery goes more smoothly. There are over 30 pier reviewed PubMed studies that conclude - Chiropractic evaluation and treatment during pregnancy may be considered a safe and effective means of treating common musculoskeletal symptoms that affect pregnant patients.

CHILDREN

This discussion has focused mainly on adult and how they experience and can benefit from chiropractic care, but do the same truths apply to children? Children are typically smaller and are still going through periods of rapid growth and development so can they benefit from chiropractic intervention? Indeed, the answer is once again an emphatic yes. Any individual who can benefit from proper alignment of the spine can benefit from some degree of chiropractic care.

Children may be subject to the same precipitating factors than can bring adults in for treatment. They may experience the same injuries or other causes of spinal misalignment and can likewise benefit from chiropractic adjustments.

Because the amount of force applied is already adjusted on a patient by patient basis, children are treated in the manner that is most suitable to them. The art of chiropractic care is individualized and transfers well to children. The application of pressure may be lessened, but the underlying principles are the same.

You may think of other special cases where you may think that the potential for chiropractic care may be questionable. You may wonder if everyone can truly benefit from chiropractic intervention. Again, the individualized nature of chiropractic treatment makes it all possible. By adjusting every treatment to the patient, chiropractic care remains as safe and as effective as possible. Anyone can benefit from correct spinal alignment so anyone who needs help in that area can benefit from chiropractic care.

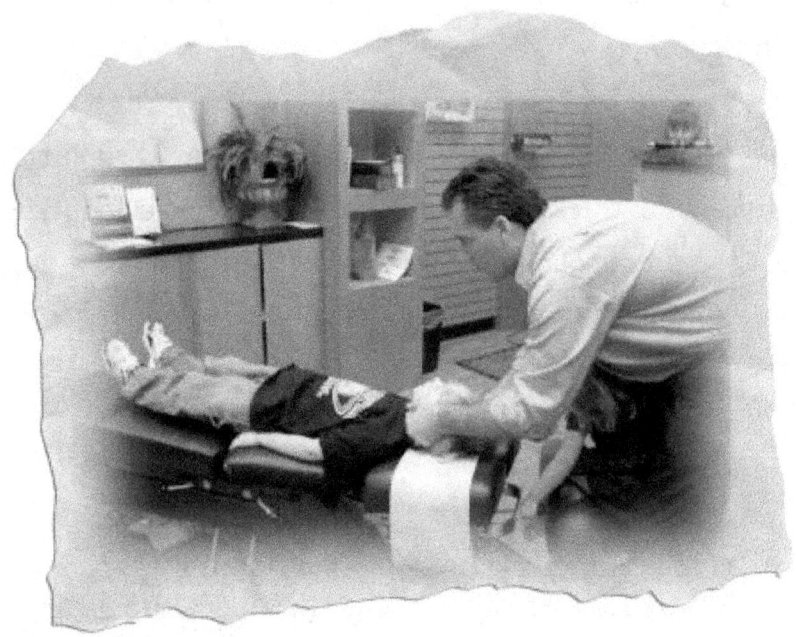

Dr. Baldasare has been certified in pediatric chiropractic adjusting since graduating from Life Chiropractic University in 1997. Here he is adjusting his son, Braxton.

4
BENEFITS OF CHIROPRACTIC CARE

"What we're here to do, as wellness experts, is not to solve a person's health problem but what creates it." - Dr. Brent Baldasare

There are many benefits that have been linked to chiropractic care. The most obvious are pain relief from acute or repetitive injuries, usually manifesting as pain in the back or as headaches, but the list does not end there.

Chiropractic care seeks to treat the cause of a problem and not just the symptoms. The benefit of this is that we get to the root of the problem. By treating the condition that causes the symptoms instead of the symptoms themselves, chiropractors can eliminate all the symptoms that the condition produces. The benefits of such an approach are extensive. It would be best to begin an understanding of the results of chiropractic care with a basic exploration of the common problems that cause patients to seek out chiropractic care and how these problems may benefit from such care.

PAIN RELIEF

The topic of pain relief covers many areas of the body. It may begin with headaches and extend to a discussion of back pain, neck pain, and joint pain. Every case is unique so only a cursory explanation can be given, but this will help you to understand the general concept and principles at work.

Back pain, for instance, is more complicated than whether you have it or not. It may be located in different parts of the back. The pain may also be a dull feeling of discomfort or a sharp pain. You must also take into consideration if the pain is a constant presence or if it only appears when certain positions are assumed.

The severity of the pain is another factor. It may be a mild feeling of discomfort, or it may be agony. The pain may exist independently or it may coexist with numbness or tingling sensations.

Pain without tingling or numbness may be caused by spinal joint inflammation, muscle tears, poor posture, or improper lumbar curve. This is not an exhaustive list, but it allows you to see how what may seem to be a simple problem could be caused by a number of different conditions. Excess weight, especially around the midsection, can contribute to postural problems and may cause or worsen back pain.

Pain with tingling may be caused by disc bulges, disc degeneration, herniated discs, or even cancer. These are only a few possible causes. Numbness or a tingling sensation is not natural in the body especially if the numbness is prolonged.

The treatment of back pain may include adjustments that seek to stretch the muscles and increase the range of motion of joints. These actions can diminish pain and any tension in the muscles while increasing a patient's mobility. The patient may also require additional therapy to strengthen the surrounding muscles, but chiropractic care alone can often reduce the patient's suffering and increase mobility.

Headaches are often thought of as a problem requiring some over the counter medication and then continuing with your day. They may, however, be caused by poor spinal alignment and can often be improved with the help of chiropractic care. They, too, can have a myriad of causes and can range from mild headaches to migraines.

The use of chiropractic care to ameliorate symptoms is often effective for patients who suffer from migraines. In some cases, muscles at the base of the neck clench and tighten which can create tension in the neck and may be a contributing factor to certain types of headaches. Chiropractic care can intervene and often provide relief from the pain and tension associated with these issues.

Neck pain can be caused by poor posture, acute trauma, or degeneration. The lack of proper posture in the work place is an increasingly seen cause of neck problems and pain problems in general. Computer screens especially cause people to put their heads into awkward positions. A computer screen that is not properly placed forces an individual to tilt their head at an awkward angle and often forces them to do so for a prolonged period of time on a daily basis. Over time, this poor positioning is bound to create problems. The weight of the head is significant and can easily strain the muscles of the neck if the weight is not distributed equally as it is when an individual's posture is correct.

Chiropractic care can help to relieve pain and restore lost range of motion in the neck, allowing the patient to return to a natural position where the head is resting upon the neck and not leaning forward placing further undue strain on the neck. To maintain these results, the faulty ergonomics of the workplace will have to be fixed.

Shoulder pain is another injury centered on a joint that may very well benefit from chiropractic intervention. These injuries are made all the more important by the fact that people use their arms constantly in daily life. Shoulder pain may be cause by tendonitis, muscle tears, ligament tears, and any other of a number of conditions.

Injuries to the shoulder tend to be caused by a clearly identifiable traumatic experience although this is not always the case. Some shoulder injuries occur without a clear precipitating event.

Chiropractic treatments for shoulder injuries can prove helpful and are often used in conjunction with other healing modalities such as massage therapy. The joint and muscles must also undergo rehabilitation as the limited use experienced after the injury will necessitate it. To work towards healing the injury and then to return as much of the former joint mobility and strength as possible will most likely require a combination of differing treatment modalities.

IMPROVED IMMUNE SYSTEM

One of the most important studies showing the positive effect chiropractic care can have on the immune system and general health was performed by Ronald Pero, Ph.D., chief of cancer prevention research at New York's Preventive Medicine Institute and professor of medicine at New York University. Dr. Pero measured the immune systems of people under chiropractic care as compared to those in the general population and those with cancer and other serious diseases.

In his initial three-year study of 107 individuals who had been under chiropractic care for five years or more, the chiropractic patients were found to have a 200% greater immune competence than people who had not received chiropractic care, and 400% greater immune competence than people with cancer and other serious diseases.

The immune system superiority of those under chiropractic care did not diminish with age. Dr. Pero stated.

"When applied in a clinical framework, I have never seen a group other than this chiropractic group to experience a 200% increase over the normal patients.

This is why it is so dramatically important. We have never seen such a positive improvement in a group..."
Pero R. *"Medical Researcher Excited By CBSRF Project Results." The Chiropractic Journal, August 1989; 32.*

The chiropractic immunology connection was strengthened in 1991 when Patricia Brennan, Ph.D. and other researchers conducted a study that found improved immune response following chiropractic treatment. Specifically, the study demonstrated the "phagocytic respiratory burst of polymorphnuclear neutrophils

(PMN) and monocytes were enhanced in adults that had been adjusted by chiropractors."

In other words, the cells that act like "Pac-Man" eating and destroying bad cells are enhanced through chiropractic care.
Brennan P, Graham M, Triano J, Hondras M. "Enhanced phagocytic cell respiratory bursts induced by spinal manipulation: Potential Role of Substance P." J Manip Physiolog Ther 1991; (14)7:399-400.

Another important study was performed at the Sid E. Williams Research Center of Life Chiropractic University. The researchers took a group of HIV positive patients and adjusted them over a six-month period. What they found was that the "patients that were adjusted had an increase of forty-eight percent (48%) in the CD4 cells (an important immune system component)." These measurements were taken at the patients' independent medical center, where they were under medical supervision for the condition. The control group (the patients that were not adjusted) did not demonstrate this dramatic increase in immune function, but actually experienced a 7.96% decrease in CD4 cell counts over the same period.

When we read the results of that study we were shocked that we hadn't heard about it earlier or that it didn't make the headline news or was on the front page of every newspaper. Those are very impressive results with important implications!

OTHER BENEFITS

The other possible benefits of chiropractic care are endless. You are not just treating one isolated part of the body when you improve the alignment of the spine. You are allowing the entire system to function more efficiently.

This is another example of the system's integrated nature. When you correct alignment of nerve signals to one part of the body, you do not just work to make better whatever condition brought that patient in for treatment in the first place. You also allow for clearer, faster signals to reach that entire region of the body.

The ability to treat isolated, discernable health conditions is a straightforward benefit of chiropractic treatment, but its effects also include a less describable improvement of the functioning of all bodily systems. Not all systems deteriorate to the point where the need for improvement is obvious. Some systems have a less discernible downward slide that may not even be noticed until their full potential is once again restored and realized.

Many benefits of chiropractic care have been observed both by science and by anecdotal evidence from patients themselves. It is true that one must take into account the possibility of a placebo effect wherein patients simply convince themselves that they are experiencing an improvement in their symptoms regardless of the efficacy of a treatment protocol, but the consistent nature of positive feedback and the research that has supported these claims is difficult to ignore. The benefits of chiropractic care for patients are very real.

You may view the ability to treat back problems, neck problems, and problems with the spine without having to resort to surgery as a major benefit of chiropractic services. Chiropractic care may not allow patients to avoid surgery in all cases, but it has allowed many to forego invasive procedures, including myself.

The word invasive is not used in this case to mean that it is entirely detrimental. Rather, surgery can do a lot of good when necessary. It is only meant that surgery by its very nature is an invasive procedure. This description separates it from chiropractic care which is non-invasive and only seeks to rearrange what is already present in the body. It works with the body in its natural form as opposed to forcibly entering the body to make alterations.

It has also been noted that the lungs may be freed up and breathing may be improved through the utilization of chiropractic adjustments. This is easily understood as chiropractic adjustments may restore the body to its correct posture which maximizes the space available for lungs to expand during each breath. A person who is hunched over may be physically restricting breathing through posture so a reversal of this postural abnormality would restore breathing capacity. Because respiratory functioning is such an important part of the overall functioning of the body, this restoration of breathing capacity can dramatically increase a person's energy and overall oxygenation – which may also result in increased protection from hormonal imbalances.

It has been noted that chiropractic care has managed to improve conditions such as the common cold, allergies, and asthma in some patients. After gaining a working knowledge of how the body works and how chiropractic care improves the state of the body as a complete entity, this is not surprising. This ability to improve numerous health afflictions is in addition to the way that this treatment has been known to aid the nervous system in its functioning as well as assisting the functioning of the heart and the coronary arteries. The effects of chiropractic care seem to go well into every system of the body in practice as well as in theory.

In our experience most patients experience a better feeling of overall health and quality of life. This may included lessened anxiety, depression, and tension. By allowing some patients to relax and improve their mood state, the effects of chiropractic treatment extend further into the promotion of an overall sense of well being. Aside from the feeling of relief that surely accompanies a reduction in pain and physical problems, these results can often be found when chiropractic care is used solely as a preventative measure.

Chiropractic care has been known to increase a patient's energy level and, of course, improve the patient's ability to heal. With all the benefits that chiropractic care can provide, it is no wonder it's the second largest of the three primary health care provider segments in the United States.

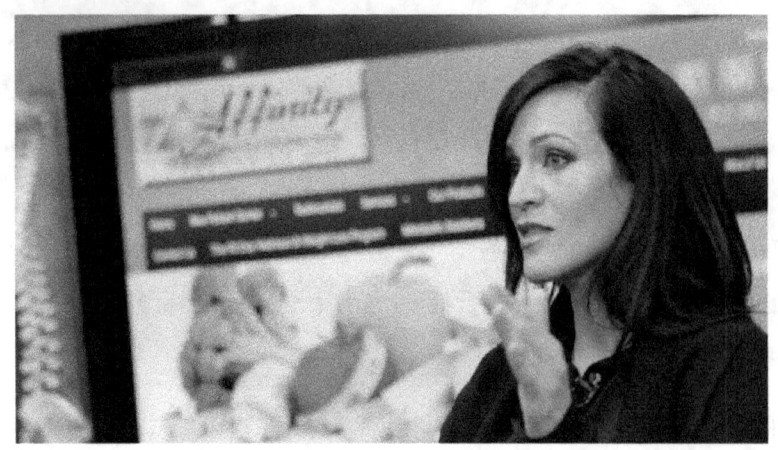

Dr. Ahitsha Ortiz is an Affinity Chiropractor that specializes in nutrition, weight loss and postural correction.

5

THE PHILOSOPHY OF CHIROPRACTIC CARE

Chiropractic care is sometimes thought of as an alternative method of dealing with health problems. The traditional methods may include the aforementioned options of medications and surgery. Both are, arguably, invasive, expensive and can depend upon artificial materials from outside of the patient's body to complete the healing process.

In most cases, a healthy body should be able to heal itself. We have a remarkable capacity for regeneration. This assumes that the body's basic needs are met and that the body is properly maintained. You would not expect a weakened body to be able to perform as well in physical activities as a healthy body so too should you not expect a body that has been weakened by spinal misalignment to be able to perform as well as a healthy body.

While physical activity may be an outward and easily recognized demonstration of inner weakness, the immune system also reflects the health of the body as a whole. If the body is not balanced and maintained then the immune system cannot work at peak efficiency. If a body were out of balance in some other way then this weakening may be more obvious to the casual observer.

If a person were malnourished, for example, you would have no problem linking all the resulting functional deficiencies and internal problems to the malnutrition. So, too, nerve function pervades the many systems, cells, and processes of the body just as proper nutrition does. You would not expect an individual's body to be as able to fight off infection if they were malnourished. Similarly, a body weakened by poor spinal alignment and diminished nerve function cannot express its full immune system potential either.

Chiropractic care has as its goal the restoration of the natural ability of the body to heal. It wishes to avoid, whenever possible, toxic or synthetic sources to aid in the healing process. For every action there is an equal and opposite reaction, this is not only true for objects in motion it's true for the chemicals we allow in our body.

Iatrogenic disease means "brought forth by the healer" or in other words death and disease caused by the treatment, most often being drugs and surgery. Last year alone over 225,000 people died of properly prescribed medication and surgery. That makes medical care the third leading cause of death in the U.S. behind cancer and heart disease.

"Chiropractic is not designed to make you instantly feel better.

Chiropractic is designed to make you instantly heal better!"

HOW IT DIFFERS FROM TRADITIONAL MEDICINE

In a nutshell, chiropractors and traditional medical doctors approach disease from opposite ends of the spectrum. The medical model believes diseases cause ill health, whereas chiropractic practitioners believe ill health leads to disease.

Traditional medical doctors have become experts at treating the body in crisis mode, when health has faltered to the point where various disease processes can take hold. Symptoms are treated with drugs and surgery, which can weaken the already compromised patient even further, allowing opportunistic infections and side effects to take their toll. The body is seen as a series of organs and tissues, instead of vital parts of a whole human being.

As chiropractors we're trained to see patients' disorders as evidence that the patient's body is out of balance, due to a variety of factors including genetic predisposition, physical and emotional habits and attitudes, and dietary and exercise deficits.

We work with the patient to correct physical imbalances through spinal manipulation and physical therapy, we also educate patients on proper diet and exercise programs.

There has traditionally been a lack of appreciation between the traditional medical establishment and the chiropractic community, but this is slowly changing. Over time the irrefutable evidence that chiropractic care works to create favorable, drug-free and natural relief from a variety of conditions has led many in the medical profession to acknowledge that there is a very valuable place for chiropractic care in the healthcare spectrum.

Traditional medicine historically has viewed the body as individual parts instead of a whole system. Treatment often begins with over-the-counter medicine, such as ibuprofen or aspirin and bed rest. If symptoms persist, treatment progresses to NSAIDs (non-steroidal anti-inflammatory drugs), prescription drugs like Naproxen, or the newer COX-2 inhibitors such as Vioxx and Celebrex.

NSAIDs come with well-known side effects like stomach irritation and ulcers, but also have some not-so-well-known side effects like swelling and increased blood pressure and the potential for liver and kidney damage (this is why your doctor may require periodic blood tests to check for liver damage). So the medical approach is to treat this biomechanical problem chemically.

Why doesn't the medical profession treat this biomechanical problem biomechanically?

Because it does not have conservative biomechanical treatments at its disposal. As was explained by Karel Lewit, MD a neurologist who is self-trained in manipulation. As stated in The Manipulative Therapy in Rehabilitation of the Locomotor System, 3rd edition Oxford England Chapter 10, ***"Disturbed mechanics or function in the musculoskeletal system is the single most common cause of pain syndromes for patients but has never formed part of the curriculum in medical education – either in undergraduate or postgraduate specialty education."***

He concludes that the chiropractic profession has grown largely because of this major gap in medical education and practice. The main treatments are specialized drugs and surgery. The medical approach is often that something is wrong with the body and must be fixed. It is sometimes believed that only those trained professionals in the medical field have the ability to fix a basically "broken" body by introducing some outside influence into the system.

For example, pain may be treated with medications, and muscle injuries may be treated through various surgical procedures. In both instances, foreign influences are used to attempt to fix problems. These techniques, while they have the best of intentions, may result in other harmful side effect to the body such as toxicity or even addictions.

Medications are artificial outside influences on the body. They may have side effects that are often difficult to predict. These adverse effects occur because the medication seeks to provide an influence that the body cannot produce or is currently unable to produce on its own.

Medications have different reactions when they are introduced into different individuals. There is not always one medication that improves a condition for every patient. Instead, there are several choices of medications that must be gone through in a process of trial and error.

Medications meant to help can have the potential to harm because their exact effects in a patient's body are unknown. Surely, there has to be a better method than attempting to give patients medication with unknown effects.

Dr. Ben Goldacre sheds some insight, in his book Bad Pharma, on how drug companies mislead doctors and harm patients by manipulating data and slanting the results in favour of the drugs they sell. When it comes to drug therapy it's "buyer beware". Some, if not most, of the information your doctor has been taught may not be in the best interest for your health, it may be in the profit for the pharmaceutical company.

10 Steps to Reduce Your Pharmaceutical Expenses Now
Take charge of your own health now instead of handing it over to the drug companies.

How do you do that?

You can start by using the Internet to locate non-drug alternatives to your health challenges. Many start with Mercola.com as it has more than 150,000 pages to help you understand more about how you can improve your health without drugs or surgery, through simple lifestyle modifications.

These are a few basic tenets of optimal health that have **always remained permanent truths**, regardless of what marvels modern science comes up with next:
1. Eat a healthy diet that's right for your nutritional type (paying very careful attention to keeping your insulin levels down)
2. Drink plenty of clean water
3. Be emotionally and mentally fit
4. Exercise

5. Get adequate amounts of Vitamin D and Omega 3
6. Limit toxin exposures
7. Consume healthy fats
8. Eat plenty of raw food & greens
9. Optimize *insulin* and *leptin* levels
10. Keep your body properly aligned and in motion

These recommendations may not always point to chiropractic care, but the philosophy extends beyond one particular method of healing. It is an ideology wherein the simplest, most natural techniques of healing are preferred over invasive techniques that can do harm even as they attempt to promote healing.

If something you were eating was making you sick then you would stop eating it. If something you did was causing you pain then you could stop doing it. You would not want to continue doing something that was harming you just because you could take a pill that would make you numb to its unpleasant effects.

In the case of pills for pain, you would still be doing damage to your system even if you could not feel it. You have not fixed the problem. You would only be hiding from it until it once again became impossible to ignore. In such cases, taking pills masks your problem instead of dealing with the cause.

Likewise, surgery is invasive. This is not to say that surgery is unnecessary or not a valuable medical tool. In many cases surgery has proven to be helpful for patients with certain conditions. However, in cases where surgery can be avoided, it surely would be a better option. Take the case of Jonathan Stelly who was playing baseball professionally, when he was told he needed a pacemaker. He stopped playing ball, but found out later he did not actually need the surgery that changed his life forever.

Jonathan Stelly was 22, a semi-pro baseball player aiming for the big leagues, when a fainting spell sent him to his cardiologist for tests. The doctor's office called afterward with shocking news: If Stelly wanted to live to age 30, he was told, he'd need a pacemaker.

Stelly knew it would be the end of his baseball dream, but he made a quick decision. "I did what the doctor said," he recalls. "I trusted him."

Months after the surgery, local news outlets reported that the Louisiana cardiologist, Mehmood Patel, was being investigated for performing unnecessary surgeries. Tens of thousands of times each year, patients are wheeled into the nation's operating rooms for surgery that isn't necessary, a USA TODAY review of government records and medical databases finds. Some, such as Stelly, fall victim to predators who enrich themselves by bilking insurers for operations that are not medically justified. Even more turn to doctors who simply lack the competence or training to recognize when a surgical procedure can be avoided, either because the medical facts don't warrant it or because there are non-surgical treatments that would better serve the patient, like chiropractic.

The scope and toll of the problem are enormous, yet it remains largely hidden. In a CBS study more than one-third of total knee replacements performed in the U.S. were deemed "inappropriate" in a new study that used a patient classification system to weigh the risks and benefits. The study found that only 44 percent of surgeries were classified as appropriate, meaning the expected benefits outweighed the likely risks for that patient.

It would seem that everyone, including surgeons, would agree that the best course of action would be to allow the body to perform its own healing in its own way and in its own time. We know the body has an innate wisdom all its own. It is a remarkable construct that has a keen awareness for what it does and does not need. Given the right circumstances, self-healing is often a distinct possibility. Chiropractic care provides those right circumstances.

This is not a dismissal of traditional medical practices but a call for re-examination of them. Are they still the best methods that medical professionals have at their disposal? Could these changes in the human body be completed in another manner? Is it time for a re-evaluation of society's very notion of the healing process?

6

WHY CHIROPRACTIC CARE MIGHT BE RIGHT FOR YOU

It may be beneficial to end with a review of the basics of chiropractic care. Chiropractic care seeks to help your body to heal itself. This perspective has been present since the beginning of recorded history. It has evolved into a science that requires thorough training for all those who wish to be licensed to practice.

Chiropractic science is based on the fact that the spine is a conduit for messages to travel to and from the brain. This is the vehicle through which the brain affects the body and through which signals are relayed back to the brain. The state of the spine can affect the entire body's ability to function.

In chiropractic care, we first evaluate a patient and that patient's spinal alignment to see if chiropractic care is a viable method of treatment for the issues at hand. If other methods of healing might be more suitable a patient may be referred to another physician or work in conjunction with chiropractic treatment.

A chiropractor applies pressure to retrain the spine to assume its proper alignment. This is the chiropractic adjustment, and it is at the heart of the physical practice of chiropractic care.

Because chiropractic care seeks to fix the circumstances that created the problems in the first place, it seeks out a lasting solution. A pill may make you feel better, but it may not fix the underlying issue. It is only by rectifying the underlying issue that a patient finds true lasting relief. This is the philosophy that underlies the practice of chiropractic treatment.

This may seem to be an alternative approach for a society that prefers instant cures, but true healing must deal with the underlying issues. True healing takes time.

Chiropractic care is not about avoiding other avenues of healing. It is about finding the most effective, natural, and least intrusive method for a patient to heal.

Chiropractic care helps your body to heal itself the natural way. You can ignore the pain or you can take a pill to make it go away, but in many cases this only avoids the matter at hand. These actions or a state of inaction will not necessarily heal the problem and may even allow your condition to get worse.

Would you want to have surgery when your body may be able to heal itself with a little help? Would you want to take a pill knowing that the problem may still be there even if you no longer feel it? Do you want a body that has the ability to heal itself?

Chiropractic care is all about natural healing. It is meant to restore the natural order that your body needs to function at its best. Because the nature of chiropractic care leads it to restore order to a system that impacts so much of your health, you may not just heal the problems that you have. You might avoid future problems and improve your overall health, and you can do it in a natural way. These are the benefits of chiropractic care.

For more information about our practice visit

www.FamilyChiropractor.com

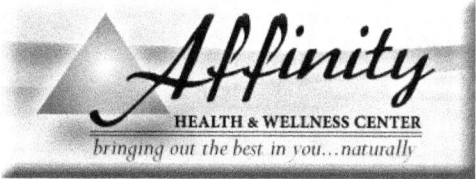